Office
Fitness Fix

Office
Fitness Fix

AN EASY 4-WEEK PLAN TO SLAM
SELF-CARE INTO YOUR WORK LIFE

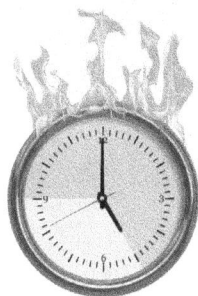

◆ ◆ ◆

LISA ZASKI

ISBN: 0692451595
ISBN-13: 9780692451595
Library of Congress Control Number: 2015912455
Lisa Zaski, Pleasant Hill, CA

Dedication

◆ ◆ ◆

This publication is a labor of love for any person who sits for hours each day in order to make a living.

To Hannah Nicole and to Joseph Alexander, my incredible children who have developed beyond my wildest expectations or dreams.
Your inner beauty, intelligence, substance and humor profoundly and positively enhance each one of my days.

Medical Disclaimer

◆ ◆ ◆

Always consult your physician before beginning any exercise program. This general information is not intended to diagnose any medical condition or to replace your healthcare professional. Consult with your healthcare professional to design an appropriate exercise prescription. If you experience any pain or difficulty with these exercises, stop and consult your healthcare provider.

Foreward

◆ ◆ ◆

IN MY DAILY PROFESSIONAL LIFE as a rheumatologist (a physician specializing in arthritis, musculoskeletal disorders, and autoimmune diseases), I see many people with back, neck, arm, and leg disorders, as well as carpal tunnel syndrome. These painful problems, which may negatively affect one's quality of life, are often the result of a sedentary lifestyle caused by the tremendous number of hours that so many of us spend sitting at a computer as part of work and leisure activities. Research shows that in addition to physical inactivity's causing significant musculoskeletal problems, it can also increase our risk of heart disease, diabetes, and cancer.

In this excellent and helpful book, *Office Fitness Fix: An Easy 4-Week Plan to SLAM Self-Care into Your Work Life*, Lisa Zaski gives us an overview of the negative impact of a sedentary life on so many aspects of our health, citing the most current medical research. More importantly, she outlines a practical, easy to follow, scientifically-based program designed to counteract the deleterious effects of spending our days and nights on a chair or couch. The exercise program is clearly outlined, accompanied by practical suggestions for using the program unobtrusively in an office environment. The SLAM program is greatly enhanced by a simple free app for one's smart phone (iPhone or Android). There is a well-proven principle that if someone incorporates an activity into his or her daily life for three weeks or more, it becomes almost "automatic." By following Ms. Zaski's four-week program, many of us will be able to increase our physical and mental health and lose weight at the same time.

I was so impressed with the office-based exercise program, accompanying app, diet suggestions, and long-term follow-up program that I have added her four-week method of SLAM self-care into my work life. I hope that you will too!

Brian R. Kaye, M.D.
Clinical Professor of Medicine
University of California, San Francisco

Table of Contents

Medical Disclaimer vii

Foreward. ix

Acknowledgments xiii

Chapter 1 Introduction. 1

Chapter 2 The Problem: "Buns of Cinnamon" 4

   -The Many Hours You Sit Each Day 4

   -Your Body's Response To So Much Sitting 7

   -Your Options For Change 15

Chapter 3 The Challenge: "No Headstands Here Please" 17

   -Better Health Through A Reminder-Based Workday 17

   -Incorporating Your Plan For Improved Health 18

   -Introducing Non-Exercise Activity Thermogenesis 19

   -Sticking With The Concept Of Moving While Working. . . .20

Chapter 4 The 4-Week Method: "Put Diamonds On Your Floor" 23

   Reminders, Timers, And Practice .27

   -Week 1. 29

   -Week 2. 39

   -Week 3. 42

   -Week 4. 44

Chapter 5 *The Long-Term Commitment:* "Hang Out With Eagles" . . .55

   -Office Fitness Fix Fuel. 55

   -Office Fitness Fix Community. 58

   A Special Note To Employers: 63

   FootNotes. 65

Acknowledgments

◆ ◆ ◆

Foreword: Dr. Brian R. Kaye, M.D.

Editor: Deborah Sosebee
Content Review: Ephraim Heller, Janell Marino, Deborah Sosebee
Cover Design Review: Hannah Gershony, Joan Diengott,
Sheila Mudd, Joseph Gershony

Office Fitness Fix Feedback from Inception to Fruition:
Georges Carantonis

CHAPTER 1

Introduction

◆ ◆ ◆

"Warning: Before beginning a program of physical
inactivity, consult your doctor. Sedentary living is
abnormal and dangerous to your health."

-FRANK FORENCICH,
Exuberant Animal: The Power of Health,
Play and Joyful Movement

MOST OF US NEED EMPLOYMENT. The great comedy writer Robert Oren once said, "Every day I get up and look through the Forbes list of the richest people in America. If I'm not there, I go to work!" Assuming that you have not quite made it to the aforementioned Forbes list, off you go each day into the world of colleagues, computers, desks and chairs. Financial demands are great in order to pay for food, housing, clothing, cars, kids, pets, recreation and vacations. Still, just because you must work to support yourself and your family does not mean that you need to sacrifice your own personal health. On the contrary, contributing to your health is *your* choice. Through proper planning and organization, improved personal health is attainable throughout each workday, right at your work desk without embarrassment or ridicule.

What does this mean exactly? *Office Fitness Fix* will teach you the value of true multi-tasking and scheduling for success. You will bridge your personal and professional goals seamlessly. Since health and wellness (to include stamina and clear-headed thinking) are fundamental for the achievement of the goals set by you and your employer, *Office Fitness Fix* will show you how movement during your workday "fixes" the very sedentary lifestyle that obliterates energy, threatens health, and sabotages success. Incorporating self-care and fitness into each day of work will benefit both you and your employer.

However, the focus of this book is more about you. Have you heard yourself thinking or saying the following?

"Between my obligations at work and home, I don't have the luxury of time for exercise."

"Am I always going to look and feel this poorly? I feel as though I am wasting my life away, day after day, just sitting at my desk in front of my computer."

"I work all day and then race to pick up the kids. I sit at work, I sit in traffic, and I sit in the carpool lane. Later, I arrive home exhausted and then sit again each evening in front of the television just to unwind and decompress."

The big question that arises is this: how can you possibly make time for exercise? The answer? You cannot. If you could, you would already have committed yourself to a yoga class that you adore and would never miss. If you could, you would already have scheduled your time after work at the gym and asked someone else to pick up your children at school. If you could, you would already have woken up an hour early each day to jog around the block. If none of this is happening, it is due to your own personal reasons (all of which fall into the "none of your business" category, and you can say that loudly and proudly).

There are a limited number of hours in each day, and we all have to manage within the time allotted to us. Those workers who do schedule the time for regular exercise are amazing, but I, unfortunately, was definitely not a member of that group. Interestingly, the most recent research in the science of "sitting sickness" indicates that regular daily exercise does not offset the damage caused by prolonged sitting; if you work all day at a desk, the health-related problems remain. The solution? Movement must be woven into each hour of our workday, whether we exercise regularly or not. The good news is that we can easily do these movement activities while we are sitting for hours on end making a living.

Office Fitness Fix fully describes what happens to your body in a sedentary job before getting into the actual program. The tendency for many readers is to skip the science and get right to the program for a quick evaluation of whether it is helpful or not. You certainly have the option to skip ahead, but there are many reasons not to. If you are serious about your health and wellbeing, take these paragraphs one at a time. Read these pages one at a time. Try not to rush this process, because the greater your comprehension of the problem, the greater the likelihood that you will fully commit yourself to the solution.

Once you understand what is chemically happening to your body and mind during your deeply rooted perch at your desk, you will want to do something about it. Once you understand how simple alerts and a built-in scheduler can trigger healthy movement at work, you will want to start planning. Once you have planned how to squeeze movement into your professional life, you will want to start moving more and more each day. What happens at the completion of all of this learning, understanding and planning? Movement will become a habit and will become second nature, and simply sitting will become boring. *Let the multi-tasking begin!*

CHAPTER 2

The Problem:
"Buns of Cinnamon"

◆ ◆ ◆

-THE MANY HOURS YOU SIT EACH DAY

JOIN US ON A TYPICAL Monday morning. Susan is an accountant who reports to work each day at 8 o'clock. She has an incredible work ethic and is rarely late. Her commitment to her clients is unmatched, but somehow, her commitment to herself is at an all-time low. She sits down at her desk and begins to check her work-related emails. After some time, her body position has not changed as she doggedly responds to questions, concerns and action items that need completing. Two hours have passed, and Susan has not moved. Perhaps she travelled to the rest room at one point. Perhaps she did not. During the third hour, Susan begins her accounting work for each of her clients until she finally decides to open her lunchbox. As if attached to her desk, Susan snacks on the foods she brought from home in order to maximize her work time (skipping her lunch break). Her lower back begins to ache. The pain from her carpal tunnel syndrome is reminding her that she really should schedule a doctor's appointment, and her neck is cramping up again.

Let us go backwards in time to see another example. At nine o'clock on that same day, the secretaries begin their work in the front office. They turn on their computers and nestle into their chairs. The first phone call of the day comes in, and off they go! The secretaries are busy, so much so that they do not even notice when the first hour of work has passed. Each dutiful secretary is answering phone calls, answering emails, greeting guests, and arranging appointments for the executives in the building, *but they have not moved from their chairs.*

Down the street is another office building. This one provides space for computer programmers. These tech-gurus will connect to your computer off-site and become "ghosts," running your machine from a remote location in order to diagnose problems as a service. What is it that these people are *not doing*? Moving!

The sedentary nature of computer-based office work can make a person wonder about its effect on our bodies. Equally important is for each person to understand the duration of time that he or she actually sits. How many hours are we concerned about here? The U.S. Bureau of Labor Statistics created a clear picture of our usage of sitting time with the following chart[1]:

"For example, the chart… shows how employed persons ages 25 to 54, who live in households with children under 18, spent their time on an average workday. These individuals spent an average of 8.7 hours working or in work-related activities, 7.7 hours sleeping, 2.5 hours doing leisure and sports activities, and 1.3 hours caring for others, including children."

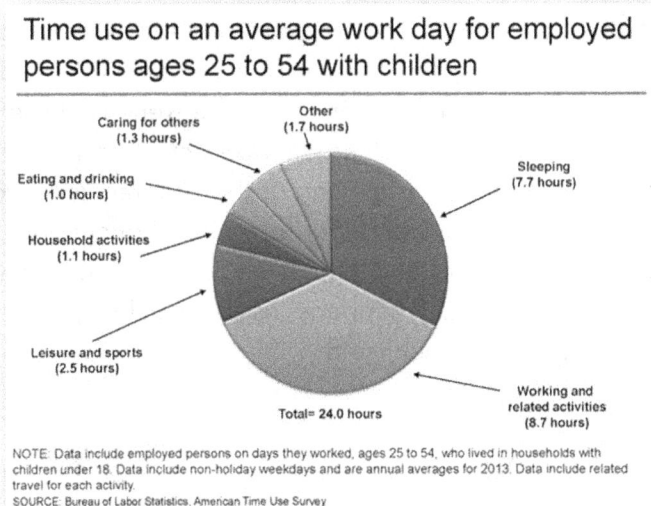

Time use on an average work day for employed persons ages 25 to 54 with children

Caring for others (1.3 hours)
Other (1.7 hours)
Eating and drinking (1.0 hours)
Sleeping (7.7 hours)
Household activities (1.1 hours)
Leisure and sports (2.5 hours)
Working and related activities (8.7 hours)
Total= 24.0 hours

NOTE: Data include employed persons on days they worked, ages 25 to 54, who lived in households with children under 18. Data include non-holiday weekdays and are annual averages for 2013. Data include related travel for each activity.
SOURCE: Bureau of Labor Statistics. American Time Use Survey

At a glance, you can see that the categories labeled "Eating and drinking," "Leisure and sports" and "Working and related activities" equate to 12.2 hours. Since you purchased this book, it might be possible that your personal "Leisure and sports" category describes *watching* sports, not really *playing* sports, and we already know what the term "leisure" means. In looking at the chart, it is not clear what the category called "Other" actually means, but it very well could be that the "Other" 1.7 hours in *your* day refers to driving, or taking public transportation, and/or watching more television. Let us cut you a break and leave out those 1.7 hours for a moment. Let us only speak of the average hours at work and the average number of sedentary hours at home as indicated in the chart. If you sit at a desk at work for seven hours each day, and if you relax in the evenings watching television or engaging in personal computer time, a conservative total would be 10 hours. Do you have a commute to work in your car or on a mode of public transportation? Do you spend any time on social media websites? Add those sitting times as well. Your sedentary behavior each day could easily add up to 11 hours. There are 24 hours in a day, and according to the Bureau of Labor Statistics, you are using 7.7 of those hours for sleep. This leaves 16.3 hours during which you are awake to use your body for conscious living. Eleven hours out of the 16.3 available hours for each business day means that as much as 68% of your awake existence during the workweek involves sitting still. In your own personal reality, does your sedentary behavior look any better on the weekends? These statistics may shock you, but *it is critical that you take action and make changes in your life*. The goal for the beginning of this program is for you to figure out your own sitting statistics. For how many hours do you sit each day? Once you have that total, I think it would be a fine time for me to introduce you to what really happens inside your body while you are doing all that sitting. Brace yourself!

-Your Body's Response To So Much Sitting
"I really don't think I need buns of steel.
I'd be happy with buns of cinnamon." –Ellen Degeneres

The result of prolonged sitting goes way beyond the cinnamon-buns joke from Ellen Degeneres! What happens when we completely lose ourselves in the din of the blue rays emanating from our computer screens? What is going on inside of us when the outside of us does not move for extended periods? Our industrialized world provides us with excellent opportunities to sit, constantly. Theaters, restaurants, automatic car-wash stations, social media and online shopping all contribute to the hours on our backsides. *Wait!* Did I just mention online shopping? What are we doing when we shop online? We are sitting. Guess what we are doing while on Facebook and Twitter and Etsy and Pinterest? We are sitting. What do we do when we pay bills and write personal notes and emails? I think you know. Excess sitting wreaks havoc on the human body, and physicians and scientists have done an excellent job reporting the findings from an enormous body of research. The list below summarizes those outcomes.

Early Death
The World Health Organization (WHO) stated in January 2015 that "*insufficient physical activity is 1 of the 10 leading risk factors for death worldwide.*" A second point of importance was that "*insufficient physical activity is a key risk factor for non-communicable diseases (NCDs) such as cardiovascular diseases, cancer and diabetes.*" [2] Did you know that prolonged sitting increases the risk of death? Did I just use the 'D' word? Unfortunately, a large amount of research has proven this fact. These relevant studies portray the excellent work done by physicians with regard to extended sitting time and human health.

For example, a report on the published scientific studies and clinical papers to which I refer was recently summarized in a press release from the University Health Network (UHN) in Toronto, Canada, *"The amount of time a person sits during the day is associated with a higher risk of heart disease, diabetes, cancer, and death, regardless of regular exercise, according to a review study published today in the Annals of Internal Medicine."* [2]

UHN and The Toronto Rehabilitation Institute, both associated with the University of Toronto, announced the findings of a research summary from 47 different studies regarding sedentary behavior. The conclusion of this decisive and extensive synopsis clearly states that prolonged sitting increases the chance of heart disease, cancer and possible death.

Here are some excerpts from the press release:

Dr. David Alter, Associate Professor of Medicine, Senior Scientist, Toronto Rehab, University Health Network (UHN), and Institute for Clinical Evaluative Sciences, University of Toronto:

"More than one half of an average person's day is spent being sedentary -- sitting, watching television, or working at a computer...Our study finds that despite the health-enhancing benefits of physical activity, this alone may not be enough to reduce the risk for disease."

*"It is not good enough to exercise for 30 minutes a day and be sedentary for 23 and half hours". In the interim, Dr. Alter underlines strategies people can use to reduce sitting time, **"The target is to decrease sedentary time by two to three hours in a 12-hour day."** [*]*

*Dr. Alter's work is supported by a career-investigator award with the Heart and Stroke Foundation, Ontario Provincial Office; and a Research Chair in Cardiovascular Prevention and Metabolic Rehabilitation at Toronto Rehab, UHN.

To be clear, the Toronto Rehabilitation Institute study demonstrates that your favorite step aerobics class would not be enough to counteract the effects of being sedentary during the rest of your day. What remains for all of us, workout mavens or not, is that we must take action and get our bodies moving, *each day, throughout the day.*

Another study from the other side of the globe reached the same conclusion. In New South Wales, Australia, researchers took data in a cross-sectional analysis of several studies involving over 220,000 Australian residents and discovered that the risk of dying early directly relates to the number of hours spent sitting down daily, unrelated to exercise habits. This study, published in the Archives of Internal Medicine, included one specific study that cut to the meat of the matter. At the conclusion of the "AusDiab" (the Australian Diabetes, Obesity, and Lifestyle Study), researchers stated the following**: "We found that having a higher number of breaks in sedentary time was beneficially associated with waist circumference, body mass index, triglycerides, and 2-h plasma glucose".** [4]

That last sentence was profound. The AusDiab directly correlated sedentary time with higher rates of serious illness and mortality, but it also found that breaking up those hours on our backsides has a direct association with improved health and wellness. Naturally, the scientific proof that waist circumference diminishes in response to a higher number of breaks in sedentary time is tremendous! Who wants a large waist circumference? *The Office Fitness Fix* program supports your effort to schedule those much-needed breaks. The 4-week method introduces the concept of taking breaks at the beginning and then slowly increasing the frequency of those breaks. Through this program, the habit of movement during your workday will become ingrained, and serious threats like *death* can be abated.

The threat of early death may sound overly dramatic. Still, there are many other serious health consequences of prolonged sitting that are equally dramatic and can lead to a life-changing illness. One critical example is heart disease.

THE CARDIOVASCULAR RISKS

When you are sedentary for long periods, your blood flow attenuates considerably. How does reduced blood flow directly affect your heart? According to a Health & Science Report in the Washington Post, dated January 20, 2014, **"Muscles burn less fat and blood flows more sluggishly during a long sit, allowing fatty acids to more easily clog the heart. Prolonged sitting has been linked to high blood pressure and elevated cholesterol, and people with the most sedentary time are more than twice as likely to have cardiovascular disease than those with the least."** [5]

Emphasizing this point, the Harvard Health Publications blog, January 29, 2014, quoted Dr. JoAnn Manson. As Chief of Preventative Medicine at Harvard-affiliated Brigham and Women's Hospital, Dr. Manson stated that **"Even if you are doing the recommended amount of moderate to vigorous exercise, you will still have a higher risk of mortality if you're spending too many hours sitting...each of these behaviors is important and has an independent effect on cardiovascular disease and mortality."** [6]

To be clear, prolonged sitting results in a reduction of blood flow. Fatty acids develop and can easily clog the heart arteries. Clogged arteries elevate blood pressure, which in turn may result in cardiovascular disease. Indeed, there is a direct line of cause and effect, and the result is quite detrimental. This might make you wonder, "Is there more to this downward spiral?" You had to ask.

THE PANCREAS AND DIABETES

In addition to the possibilities of early death and cardiovascular disease, diabetes represents another likely outcome of prolonged sitting. One of the organs in the human body is the pancreas, which is critical to the digestive system. The pancreas has two vital roles, one being the exocrine system to aid in digestion, and the other being the endocrine system to produce insulin and regulate blood sugar. With regard to diabetes, insulin allows muscle cells to take up sugar from the bloodstream that was absorbed from food. According to the American Journal of Clinical Nutrition via Dr. Gabe Mirkin, ***"Resting muscles pull virtually no sugar from your bloodstream, and insulin is required for the little amount of sugar the muscles use. Contracting muscles can draw large amounts of sugar from the bloodstream and do not even need insulin to do so. People who do not move their muscles have much higher blood sugar levels than those who exercise, so they are at increased risk for weight gain, diabetes, heart attacks, strokes, cancers, and premature death."*** [7]

When you remain seated for a long time, the cells that are present in the idle muscles are not reactive to the insulin production. In response to this inaction, the pancreas *increases* its production of insulin and as a result, you develop the risk of diabetes along with other diseases. The insulin response is reduced considerably after just one day of prolonged sitting. According to the Toronto Rehabilitation Institute, University Health Network (UHN) review cited earlier, the biggest health hazard stemming from prolonged sitting was a 90 percent higher risk of developing type 2 diabetes.

The *Office Fitness Fix* 4-week method includes large-muscle-group contraction. The program describes how simply standing or moving at or near your desk on a regularly-timed basis offers the break in sedentary behavior that you *physically need*. Muscle contraction and movement will draw sugar from your bloodstream in order to offset the damage done by idle muscles during the times you are seated. Still, understanding all of the risks of so much work in front of a computer screen is paramount to securing this much-needed commitment to change. Shall we move southward?

COLON CANCER

Colon cancer has been closely associated with high blood sugar and insulin levels. One study, published June 16, 2014 in the *Journal of the National Cancer Institute,* supports the opinion of Dr. Graham Colditz, the

Associate Director for Prevention and Control at Washington University's Siteman Cancer Center in St. Louis. Dr. Colditz stated, ***"High blood sugar and high insulin is a clear sort of pathway to colon cancer, and we know from intervention studies that walking lowers insulin and getting up after meals lowers blood sugar compared to sitting."*** [8]

Can you get cancer just from sitting excessively? The answer is yes. In 2010, The American Journal of Epidemiology reported the results of a study that linked the two directly. The research stemmed from the same population-based case-controlled study in Western Australia mentioned previously: ***"In this study, we found that participants who spent the most time in sedentary work had a risk of distal colon cancer that was 2 times higher than those who spent the most time in a job requiring light activity. Similarly, participants who spent 10 or more years in sedentary work had almost twice the risk of distal colon cancer and almost 1.5 times the risk of rectal cancer, of those who did not do any sedentary work."*** [9]

Regular movement lowers insulin levels and blood-sugar levels to block that "clear sort of pathway to colon cancer" that Dr. Colditz mentioned above. Regular movements, at your desk or in your workplace, step up natural antioxidants that extinguish free radicals and other potentially cancer-causing agents.

Despite the collective results of all the studies on sitting sickness, many readers might find the concern of serious illness and death to be too far in the future to worry about today. Nonetheless, the fact that you decided to read this book probably indicates that you have some level of concern. Perhaps you are experiencing some office-related maladies that affect your life right now. Are you feeling tired? Have you gained weight over the last few years? Blame those current problems on sluggish lipoprotein lipase enzymes…

FATIGUE: METABOLIC AND BIO-CHEMICAL RESPONSE

Prolonged sitting leads to incredible fatigue and low energy. To emphasize this point, Dr. Joan Vernikos, the former Director of the Life Sciences

Division of NASA and the author of *Sitting Kills, Moving Heals* describes her intensive research on gravity and the impact gravity has on our health. Working against gravity (i.e. standing, walking and lifting) actually provides benefits to the body. Simply standing up at your desk causes you to interact with gravity, forcing the activation of lipoprotein lipase enzymes. Lipoprotein lipase enzymes attach themselves to the fat in your bloodstream and transport that fat into the muscle, converting it into fuel. With prolonged sitting, there is a reduction of lipoprotein lipase enzymes, which results in low energy. As explained by Dr. Vernikos, " when you sit, especially for prolonged periods, you are not interacting with gravity. Incorporating movement while at your desk will get your blood pumping to oxygenate your cells, which in turn combats fatigue and low energy levels."[10]

WEIGHT GAIN AND MIDSECTION SPREAD

Now here is the one everyone notices right away: weight gain! Without movement, the enzymatic activity drops. Metabolism tanks. Calories are not burning and high levels of sugar remain in our blood. The result? Weight gain. The unfortunate truth about weight gain, however, is that it does not stand alone; weight gain allies itself with muscle degeneration in the abdomen, leading to a "jelly belly" and a very soft middle (just when you thought things could not get worse). Inactivity physiology, the function of an organism or its parts during the state of being sedentary, has a direct correlation with weight gain and muscle degeneration. When inactivity goes up, your weight increases and your muscles get softer. To prove the point, researchers from Tel Aviv University (TAU) concluded that **"Sitting too much causes fat cells of the buttocks to expand and stiffen, promoting obesity."** The TAU study proved that when you are sitting, the fat cells in your posterior respond to chronic pressure, leading a person to experience a faster growth of fat mass. [11]

Thankfully, the *Office Fitness Fix* method fights weight gain. The program tells you precisely how many calories you will burn each day via the movement schedule. As the frequency of alerts to move increases, so does the calorie burn. By Week 4, you will be burning 150-300 extra calories each day at work*, depending on your weight and exertion. When calculated over the period of a year, the expected weight loss could be 15 pounds, and possibly a little over 20 pounds. I imagine that the last ten pounds you gained did not appear on your body overnight. The only real achievable weight loss that has a prayer of "sticking" is the kind that is lost through a healthy change of habits. There are specific movement exercises in this book to provide you with comprehensive calorie burn or "calories out"; likewise, there is a separate chapter entitled "Office Fitness Fix Fuel" that will address your long-standing challenge with your diet, or "calories in."

The entire discussion about early death, diabetes, cancer, fatigue and weight gain might be lost on you if you are in the throes of serious pain. Chronic pain is awful. Chronic pain is debilitating and is exacerbated by long hours in front of a computer. Is it possible that regular movement exercises could help in this regard? Yes.

*based on the "yellow activity" scale, **Move A Little, Lose A Lot**, James A. Levine, MD,   PhD and Selene Yeager

Spine, Neck, Hips, Back, and Other Impacted Areas

Not only was our body not designed to be sedentary, but our minds were not designed this way either. "Foggy Brain" describes the brain's response to a low blood and oxygen supply. With regular movement of your muscles and limbs throughout each day, a renewed source of blood and oxygen to the brain prompts the release of brain chemicals, leading to brighter thinking and enlightened mood. When we settle in our chairs for hours on end, everything slows, including brain function.

That same lack of blood flow directly affects organs to be sure, but the lack of movement wreaks even more havoc on bones. If you currently spend your workday at a desk, more than likely you have already suffered from a sore neck and back, aching hips and spine. A significant lack of blood circulation also results in the obvious: the onset of deep vein thrombosis starts with swollen ankles and varicose veins, but the worst of it ends with dangerous blood clots.

There is no weight-bearing resistance when we sit. Bodily movement (walking, running and even standing) stimulates hip and lower-body bones to grow strong, and it increases the thickness and density of those bones. Any internet search into osteoporosis will return the direct correlation between osteoporosis and inactivity. Along with those sore and weak bones comes the obvious: the act of prolonged sitting results in body pain, herniated discs, nerve problems and painful joints. A seated position is physically stressful on the human body.

The breaks called for in the *Office Fitness Fix* program provide action in the large-muscle groups while providing relief for the muscles of the spine and neck. Additionally, the *Office Fitness Fix* method allows time for stretching exercises that will assuage the tightness associated with a sedentary professional life. Taking a break from an unnatural sitting position on a regular schedule can start the process of healing. This is long overdue.

-YOUR OPTIONS FOR CHANGE

The descriptions in Chapter 2 of the biochemical breakdown and deterioration of the body while you endure a full day of deskwork make clear the need for action. We have covered the primary reasons why prolonged sitting is bad for your physical and mental health. We have seen that when the electrical and enzyme activity levels in your muscles decline, there is a waterfall of perilous biochemical results. Insulin efficiency plummets, which increases the risk of diabetes, cardiovascular disease and cancer. The weight gain around your mid-section and backside is due to the sluggish enzymes that fail to break down lipids. To make matters worse, triglyceride levels drop, bringing the levels of good cholesterol (HDL) down with them. We have also noted that even regular exercise does not spare a person from the ills of extended sitting throughout each workday. No matter if you go to the gym every morning, prolonged sitting during the rest of your day damages and kills.

The answers are clear. If you are not moving, your blood is not pumping, your muscles are not stretching, your bones are not benefitting from exertion, and there are fewer engaged, challenged, and activated enzymes working for you at a bio-chemical level. The human design allows us to move, to stretch, to grasp, to bend, and to stride. You *must* move more often during the time that you sit, because your body in motion is precisely how your body thrives.

Still, how in the world do you move in an office environment while you are practically chained to a desk?

Some suggestions have come from scientists and nutritionists and doctors who have all encouraged us to "take the stairs, don't take the elevators." Unfortunately, despite those suggestions, you arrive each day at the elevator and thoughtlessly push that button for another easy ride of non-sweat activity. What are the other suggestions you have heard? "Walk for 15 minutes during lunchtime." Well, it is raining/snowing/I brought lunch from home/I have the wrong shoes/I'll start this tomorrow... We all know that common sense alone is not getting us to move. This battle against sitting sickness requires a formal plan of attack. The confusion and lack of motivation to fight the effects of prolonged sitting must be replaced by a concise method and support. The good news? A formal plan to adopt these healthy habits is now in your hands. Do you have options for change? You absolutely do.

CHAPTER 3

The Challenge:
"No Headstands Here Please"

◆ ◆ ◆

-Better Health Through A Reminder-Based Workday

In my own office experience, I was fortunate to have a private office, but it hardly felt private when my co-workers popped in for a quick question or concern. Had I been performing a headstand with my feet against the wall for a quick blood rush to my brain for inspiration, well, that would have been nothing short of embarrassing, especially if a skirt was part of my wardrobe selection that day!

To repeat, *Office Fitness Fix* does not promote any physical activity that would cause ridicule or embarrassment, headstands included. However, avoiding embarrassment does not translate to a free pass toward a sedentary professional life. Discreet self-care in the office environment results in a total win-win for both you and your employer. Your employer wins because the short physical breaks that will go practically unnoticed will provide you with increased energy at work, which in turn, will make you more productive. You win because you will feel better and you will have the peace of mind that you are warding off the ill effects of a sedentary life. If weeks, months and years have been flying by without any consideration of your own self-care each day at work, it is time to claim ownership of your health. Your employer is responsible for overseeing your work, but you alone are responsible for overseeing *you*. You can do this! The *Office Fitness Fix* program provides the framework of gradually building the habit of movement into your workday. Starting on Day 1, you can relax in the security that the personally set "habit reminders" will trigger your mind so that your body will take action. The habit reminders increase in number over time, with the goal of creating stealth exercise movement at your desk on a regular schedule. The movements suggested in *Office Fitness Fix* are exercises that you can do without fear of an awkward situation, and without having to cease when a co-worker steps into your professional space.

This is a "work-in" (not a workout) plan. You are experiencing your work-in, right at your desk, and you are warding off many negative physical maladies that would otherwise be coming your way. Certainly, that ten-pound loss mentioned previously will occur if all other factors in your life remain constant. However, if you were to incorporate a healthier eating plan and more movement on the weekends, your weight loss will increase significantly and your health will improve.

For your battle against a sedentary work life, this program provides the biggest weapon in your arsenal: the *Office Fitness Fix* Interval Timer. This free application is available on both Google Play (Android) and the Apple App Store (iPhone). This indispensable timing tool allows you to perform your work, fully concentrating on your professional tasks, and signals when to begin and end the movement exercises. As promised, these exercises are movements of which only you will be aware. The timers and reminders may be set on a low volume or even vibrate-only so that no interruptions occur during your business meetings.

-INCORPORATING YOUR PLAN FOR IMPROVED HEALTH

Your plan for movement throughout your workday is going to be three-quarters input from *Office Fitness Fix* and one-quarter input from you, based on your own professional reality. The plan outlined in Chapter 3 of this book offers systematic guidelines for incorporating enzyme-stimulating, muscle-contracting moves that will get your blood flowing and your energy levels charged at regular intervals each business day. However, your reality in your own office space will dictate how far you can take each of these steps.

Are you in a cubicle with some version of private space? Are you in an open- design office with numerous co-workers all around you? Are you in a private office with co-workers dropping by unexpectedly? All of these scenarios will work with the *Office Fitness Fix* program, but the degree to which you exercise your own creativity for movement and blood flow will depend on what you deem to be comfortable. No one, not even your employer, need know what you are doing. You will not need special permission for the moves described in this book. However, if you are lucky enough to have a private office, or even a home office, there are obviously fewer concerns about your movement activities. For those with private offices or those working at home, the *Office Fitness Fix* Community Newsletter* offers an ongoing review of advanced equipment,

information on joining the Office Fitness Fix Community may be found at www.officefitnessfix.com from exercise bands to treadmill desks, to help you tailor an expanded methodology to your own movement routine. These items are truly for the person who works solo or is lucky enough to be in a supportive office environment where movement and exercise at work are encouraged. Regardless, all of us who suffer from extended sitting times will benefit from the plan outlined in this book.

-INTRODUCING NON-EXERCISE ACTIVITY THERMOGENESIS
"My idea of exercise is a good brisk sit." - Phyllis Diller

Who knew that in 1986 Phyllis Diller was not only a comedian but also a soothsayer? Back then, the "brisk sit" comment brought loads of laughs, but today, the concept has quite the literal application. The active physiology of "brisk sitting" is part of a greater concept called non-exercise activity thermogenesis. As explained by endocrinologist Dr. James A. Levine, M.D., PhD. of The Mayo Clinic, Rochester, MN, **"Non-exercise activity thermogenesis (NEAT™) is the energy expended for everything we**

do that is not sleeping, eating or sports-like exercise. It ranges from the energy expended walking to work, typing, performing yard work, undertaking agricultural tasks and fidgeting. Even trivial physical activities increase metabolic rate substantially and it is the cumulative impact of a multitude of exothermic actions that culminate in an individual's daily NEAT." [12]

Dr. Levine investigated the concept of non-exercise activity thermogenesis and led a vast amount of research over a 20-year period with a focus on sitting disease. Dr. Levine's books *Get Up! Why Your Chair is Killing You,* and, *Move a Little, Lose A Lot: How NEAT Science Reveals How to Be Thinner, Happier, and Smarter* show the direct correlation between prolonged sitting and the decline of good health. Further described, exercise is the activity you purposefully do to promote good health. Exercise often involves going to the gym or energetically walking for 30 minutes, lifting weights or playing tennis. Exercise is exercise. On the other hand, non-exercise includes the list of activities we all do throughout the course of our day: running the vacuum, washing the car, even setting the dinner table.

Through non-exercise activity thermogenesis, we thoughtlessly yet purposefully burn calories during our daily routines. Dr. Levine's research demonstrates that if a person increases his NEAT expenditure each day, that person would burn more calories, energize enzymatic processes, and ward off major illnesses. The *Office Fitness Fix* program combines the methodology of Dr. Levine's suggestions with a concise, gradual plan of attack to increase the calorie burn of NEAT-related movements.

-STICKING WITH THE CONCEPT OF MOVING WHILE WORKING
How do you take on this program and incorporate it into your daily life? How do you stick with it in the long term? Is this going to be another passing fad? What do you actually gain by going through this program?

An Appreciation of Your Time

One of the best parts of incorporating *Office Fitness Fix* into your work life is that you gain a new appreciation for time. A commitment toward movement during each workday results in an appreciation of the time you have devoted to your own self-care. Sitting like a lump without movement begins to feel foreign, and you will actually find that you want to use your time effectively by incorporating these positive ways of taking care of yourself. In contrast, you begin to feel the loss of time when you simply sit without movement, while not achieving any personal benefits. It begins to feel like a waste of time to sit in a sedentary way. This new appreciation for time spreads to other parts of your life; you will find that the time spent shopping, cooking, and cleaning represent other wonderful opportunities for movement so that you can keep those biochemical processes in your body on full alert. This is your life; increased energy, revitalized thinking, and improved physical health all work in concert in order for you to live it!

A Respect for Your Health

Another wonderful benefit of the *Office Fitness Fix* program is an enhanced reverence for your mental and physical health. Your work life is a part of your life; it is certainly not your *whole life*! Leo Tolstoy once said, **"In the name of God, stop a moment, cease your work, and look around you."** If you took a moment to glance away from your computer and consider your own personal entity from time to time, a feeling of surprise may grab you. This is *you* sitting there, not a machine. This is you. This is about your mental and physical health. When you begin a program like *Office Fitness Fix*, you begin to acknowledge that human capacity can be devoted to both professional work and self-care. The Lamborghini will not run if you neglect its engine. Your good health, both mental and physical, is the engine that permits you to sit and work so diligently for your employer. Appreciating your health means that you care about both.

A BALANCED APPROACH TO YOUR LIFE

Giving almost everything to your employer all day is one factor. Leaving work and devoting yourself to your family is another factor. Sitting on the couch for mental and physical recuperation at the end of the day is a third factor. Let us say that you begin the *Office Fitness Fix* program tomorrow. In truth, even if you decide to relax at the day's end in order to unwind, you will at least have the peace of mind that you indeed exercised self-care throughout your workday and deserve this rest. Not surprising, the balance you feel at the end of each day for having stimulated blood flow via these self-care techniques is habit forming. Striving for balance will become your habit, even in the evenings at home.

Our non-exercise activity thermogenesis guru, Dr. Levine, described his transformation from being a heavier person to a leaner person, solely through the increase of NEAT activities. When asked what the impact of increased NEAT movements meant to his life, Dr. Levine stated, "It's like I came alive!"

Now it is your turn…

CHAPTER 4

The 4-Week Method: "Put Diamonds On Your Floor"

◆ ◆ ◆

CHANGE IS HARD. FORMING NEW habits and sticking to them is especially hard. For this reason, *Office Fitness Fix* focuses on the slow development of rock-solid changes in your professional habits in order to ameliorate your personal health. Gone are the seven to eleven hours of sedentary nothingness every single day. Over the four weeks of this plan, you will develop new habits that you can stick to by slowly incorporating the movement activities into your normal workday.

At first glance, the *Office Fitness Fix* plan may seem too easy. It is not. The exercises are easy enough to do, and you will certainly do these exercises in a better and stronger way each time you do them. The challenge, however, is not the exercise. The challenge is to incorporate movement at work, each day and each hour, at your desk. Adopting these new habits and locking them in to the manner in which you work will be the focus. Everything else, to include calorie burn and enhanced health, will follow naturally.

Surprisingly, the *biggest* challenge is to remember to set your *Office Fitness Fix* Interval Timer app at the beginning of the day or week and to remember to start this alert system every time you settle into your chair. In testing the methodology of the 4-week program, I originally had a difficult time remembering to set my own timer because I was so hell-bent on getting my work done, but finally, the timer prevailed. Perhaps your memory is better than mine (I hope so), but what eventually worked for me was to place a "Start Your Timer" note directly on my keyboard each time I rose from my chair. That way, when I settled back into my chair, I could not type a thing without seeing the note, and I never failed to set my timer again. Sheesh! We do whatever it takes.

The first week of the plan requires that you set your alert for a 60-minute interval. This commitment incorporates movement exercises for five of those 60 minutes each hour at your desk during Week 1. It might be safe to say that you would never think to do these movements without your alert system, so the alert system is critical to the program. Giving yourself an entire workweek to create this new habit is paramount to your success in the weeks to come.

As mentioned, the 4-week method addresses many health concerns, but weight loss seems to be the top priority for many. In that regard, movement in the program during Week 1 burns 625 calories in the collective five workdays. Those 625 calories burned may result in an eight-pound reduction by the end of the year if you were to continue at that level for an entire 12 months. The primary goal for Week 1, however, is to become accustomed to moving while working; losing weight is simply an added bonus to your resultant enhanced health. Certainly, the calorie count is dependent on how much you weigh and how hard you push the exercises, but 625 calories burned for Week 1 represents a conservative estimate based on movement throughout a seven-hour workday plus the exercises that follow restroom and lunch breaks. Are you seated for more than seven hours at work each day? If the answer is yes, count on additional healthy results.

By Week 4, a person on the plan will burn an average of up to 1,500 calories in a similar five-day period. Take those calories per week and multiply them by 50 weeks in a year (allowing for two weeks of vacation time), and the calories burned may result in 20 pounds lost by the end of one year. This is the idea and the goal for weight management. This is also the idea behind non-exercise activity thermogenesis. The more you move throughout each day, the easier it is to manage your weight.

The last ten pounds you gained crept up on you gradually. Losing pounds slowly is the best and most natural way for permanent change in weight and therefore health. Along with this slow calorie burn are the other benefits of increased enzymatic activity, decreased levels of sugar in the blood, and a true rest for your neck, hips, and spine. By burning calories each hour, even if those calories seem few at first, the cumulative effect of this calorie burn will aid in your weight-management goals while simultaneously battling serious illness.

> "If God wanted me to exercise, he would
> have put diamonds on my floor."
>
> - JOAN RIVERS

I am truly sorry but I cannot put diamonds underneath your desk to entice you to move! This one is on you, so let us get started. The goal for Week 1 is to get the new habit of *moving while working* so ingrained in your mind that you will become accustomed to the triggers. Setting the timer to go off only once each hour seems like nothing. Following the movement exercises for only five minutes each hour seems like nothing. *However, it is something, I assure you.* Presently, established work habits dominate your days. Adopting a new habit, even one that reminds you to move for only five minutes once an hour, presents a great challenge until you actually try it, live it, and experience it. After the first week, graduation to Week 2 requires new settings for the alert system; the alert will sound every 30 minutes instead of every 60 minutes. The following chart depicts the steady progression of increased activity throughout the four weeks:

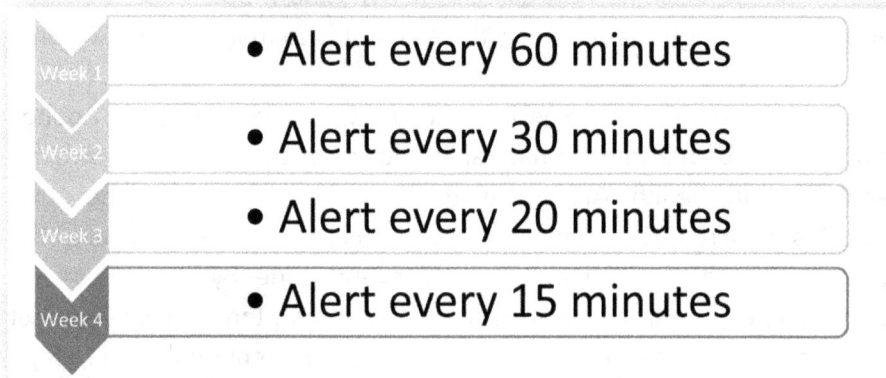

Week 1	• Alert every 60 minutes
Week 2	• Alert every 30 minutes
Week 3	• Alert every 20 minutes
Week 4	• Alert every 15 minutes

Whatever you do, do not be afraid of Week 4! When the time comes to switch your reminder to every 15 minutes, the increased calorie burn, increased energy and improved health will be the reward. Additionally, **the movement breaks provide the least amount of disruption to productivity and workflow**, so be brave and forge ahead. Your joint pain and stiffness will improve. You will thwart the chances of serious illness. Most importantly, the benefits of this slow progression of habit-changing activities over the four weeks **will provide real change**.

Let us review what the progressive track looks like:

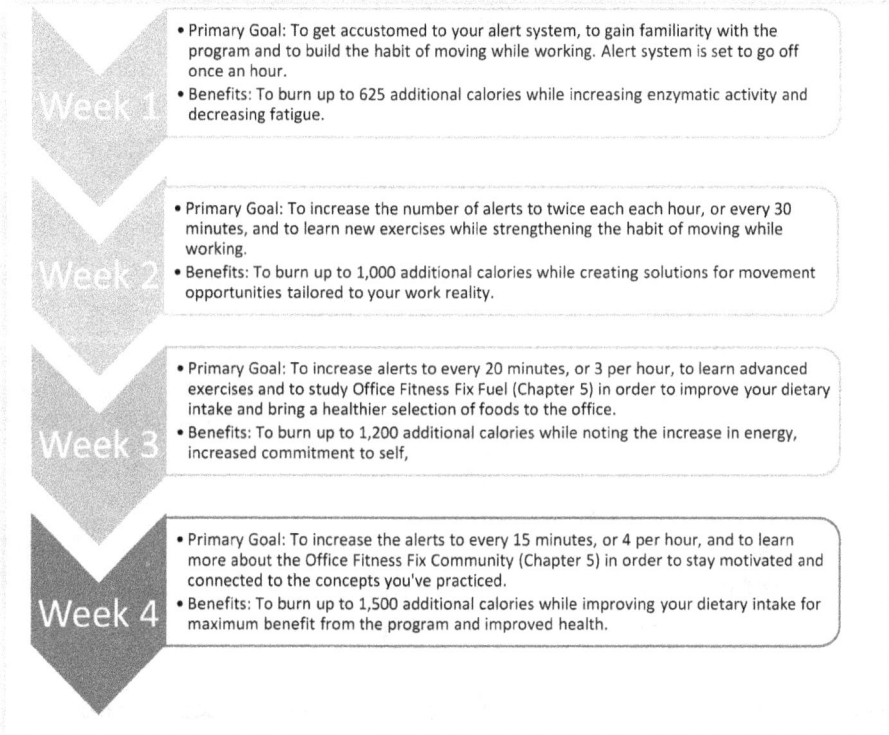

Week 1
- Primary Goal: To get accustomed to your alert system, to gain familiarity with the program and to build the habit of moving while working. Alert system is set to go off once an hour.
- Benefits: To burn up to 625 additional calories while increasing enzymatic activity and decreasing fatigue.

Week 2
- Primary Goal: To increase the number of alerts to twice each each hour, or every 30 minutes, and to learn new exercises while strengthening the habit of moving while working.
- Benefits: To burn up to 1,000 additional calories while creating solutions for movement opportunities tailored to your work reality.

Week 3
- Primary Goal: To increase alerts to every 20 minutes, or 3 per hour, to learn advanced exercises and to study Office Fitness Fix Fuel (Chapter 5) in order to improve your dietary intake and bring a healthier selection of foods to the office.
- Benefits: To burn up to 1,200 additional calories while noting the increase in energy, increased commitment to self,

Week 4
- Primary Goal: To increase the alerts to every 15 minutes, or 4 per hour, and to learn more about the Office Fitness Fix Community (Chapter 5) in order to stay motivated and connected to the concepts you've practiced.
- Benefits: To burn up to 1,500 additional calories while improving your dietary intake for maximum benefit from the program and improved health.

REMINDERS, TIMERS, AND PRACTICE

In order to get these habits to stick, you will need only two things: the *Office Fitness Fix* Interval Timer app, which is free, and *practice*. Remember Dr. Alter's suggestion from Chapter 2? He stated, ***"The goal is to decrease sedentary activity by two to three hours in a 12-hour day."*** By the end of Week 4, you will have decreased your sedentary activity by 20 minutes each hour. If, for example, you typically sit at your desk for seven hours each day, you will have decreased your sedentary time by 140 minutes, or two hours plus 20 minutes.

Still, there is so much more that you can do. Suggestions at the end of the Week 1 section include sneaking in some additional movement exercises following your trips to the restroom and on your lunch break. If you add in your restroom-break movement (no pun intended, I am talking about exercise, not anything personal), your lunch-break movement, and any additional movement you can squeeze in during the day, three hours of increased activity per day is quite achievable. Imagine, three hours less of sedentary behavior every single workday. That equals 15 hours each workweek of truly bringing your body back to life!

There is not a "price to pay" here. You are not sacrificing a thing; you are only gaining enormous health benefits to offset cancer, diabetes, heart disease and ongoing weight gain. If you follow the 4-week plan precisely as described, you will have the best chance of reversing the very processes that enticed you to buy this book in the first place. Better yet, continuing the program beyond Week 4 via support from the *Office Fitness Fix* Community (Chapter 5) will keep you motivated and on track for your own health success story.

Once you learn the exercises each week, you will spend less time thinking of them. Throughout the four weeks and beyond, you will only have to remember one word: **SLAM.** What is SLAM?

SLAM is an acronym for the order of your exercises during each movement break:

- S   Stand (to include Steps and Squats)
- L   Legs (to include Glutes and Hips)
- A   Arms (to include Neck and Shoulders)
- M Midsection (to include the Spine)

Repeat this now: "**SLAM**: **S**tand, **L**egs, **A**rms, **M**idsection" No matter which week you happen to be in, the *minutes* spent on SLAM remain the same. SLAM lasts exactly five minutes during each movement break. The order of SLAM always remains the same. The exercises within any SLAM segment are interchangeable, and for the purposes of your learning curve, new exercises each week fend off boredom and encourage creativity. The list of discreet exercises for each part of the SLAM system are so easy that, once learned, you will have them in your mind "on the ready" each time your alert system sounds. All that you will need to do is think "SLAM" and then begin the exercises in the order **Stand-Legs-Arms-Midsection.**

-WEEK 1

As mentioned previously, the *Office Fitness Fit* Interval Timer is an alert system to trigger the onset of exercise. The Interval Timer will alert you to the times when you start and when you stop your movement activities.

Relying on yourself to watch a clock may seem easy enough, but you and I both know that interruptions, phone calls, meetings, and emails are highly distractive and often make this commitment to movement an impossibility. The interval timer does the thinking for you, and best of all, it is free on the Android/Google Play and iPhone markets. The alert system suits your work lifestyle with the least amount of disruption as possible, to both the workplace environment and your co-workers.

A piece of advice: stay glued to your alert system. Your alert system tethers you to the commitment toward your own health and vitality. Never allow the alert system to come in second at the beginning of your workday. It must always come in first. Before you take a call, answer an email, or greet a guest, you must make sure that your alert system is set and that it will go off at the prescribed time.

Time to look at that timer!

Once you download the free app on your Android, iPhone or office computer, open the app and set the timer for Week 1 by doing the following:

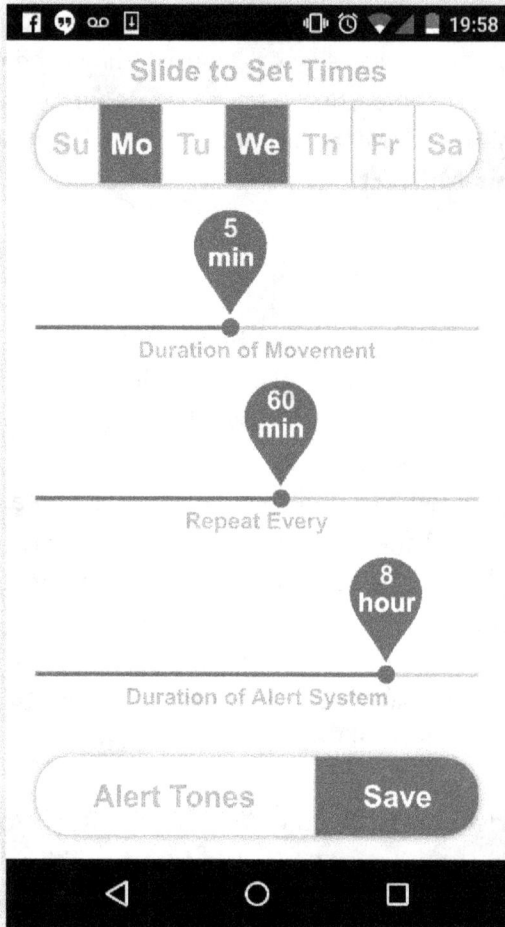

1. Choose the weekdays Monday through Friday.
2. For the "Duration of Movement" setting, set the slider at five minutes.
3. For the "Repeat Every" setting, set the slider according to the plan that particular week. Week 1, for example, requires that you set the timer for 60 minutes, which means you will take a movement break once an hour.
4. The "Duration of Alert System" is set according to your work reality. If you always begin your day at eight o'clock and take you

lunch break at noon, you may set this tab for four hours so that the interval alerts will occur four times before lunch. Once you return from lunch, set this slider according to the number of work hours you have left in your day.

5. Press the "Save" button to save your settings. Pressing "Save" initiates the countdown timer to your first movement break.

6. Here comes the fun part: choose a ring tone! There are a number of free tones available for you use, ranging from quiet tones to ones that are more aggressive if your office environment tends to be noisy. If over time you decide to expand your ring-tone selection (for kicks, as my Dad would say), you may do so for a small payment of 99 cents.

Once the Interval Timer is set and alerts you to move, each five-minute movement break consists of the SLAM order of exercises.

For SLAM, each segment receives the following time allotment:

S Stand (steps, squats) = **2 minutes**
L Legs (glutes, hips) = **2 minutes**
A Arms (neck, shoulders) = **30 seconds**
M Midsection (spine) = **30 seconds**

When you look at the SLAM time allocation, you might wonder why there is a greater percentage of time allocated to S and L. There are, of course, scientific studies behind this formula. The best and easiest way to stimulate enzymatic activity is to engage the large-muscle groups of the legs. Standing, stepping, squatting, and the leg exercises achieve just that. The remaining exercises offer relief and rest for your body. Your body will thank you.

To repeat, each SLAM movement break lasts five minutes in total. If you have the grace of time or the opportunity to make your movement break last longer than five minutes, fantastic! However, the main idea is to get your metabolic processes in gear for at least five minutes during the allotted break.

Now, the exercises!

Week 1 is such an exciting moment for you. You have finally decided to take control of your health in the most time-expedient way possible. The focus of Week 1 is to commit yourself to the alert system via the *Office Fitness Fix* Interval Timer app, and to become familiar with the following SLAM exercises. Keep in mind that these are ideas that you may take and expand upon, depending on your levels of creativity and capability. A full description of the exercises appears at the end of this chapter for easy reference.

The S Part of SLAM: Standing (to include Steps and Squats)

The S portion of the SLAM exercises is actually the same in Week 1 as it is in Weeks 2, 3 and 4. The recommendations from recent medical research mirrors the *Office Fitness Fix* program, particularly the need for us to break up extended sit times with standing. Each time your alert goes off (indicating that it is time to get up from your chair) IMMEDIATELY STAND. Tense and squeeze both thigh muscles for a few seconds, then release those muscles. Next, place the majority of your weight on the right leg and squeeze the right thigh muscle. Repeat the same on the left leg.

Now comes the creative part. For the next minute, your goal is to take some steps and squat down as many times as you can comfortably and discreetly. I emphasize "discreetly" because the *Office Fitness Fix* program is a private affair between you and your health. Making an exercising spectacle of yourself in front of your co-workers is not the goal here. Look around your office. Find ways within your office environment that allow you to squat down naturally to perform a professional task. Creative solutions might include:

- Squat down and reach for something under your desk, using your desk for support if necessary.

- Open and close the bottom drawer of a file cabinet to look for a particular file. (You might in fact want to put your most critical files in that drawer so that you will always have a reason to squat down to obtain them).
- Check the paper supply of the bottom drawer of your copy machine.

If you look around your office, you can find creative solutions to the Stand, Step and Squat segment of your movement activity. Regardless of what creative ideas you find to squat down in your office, the goal is to **take as many steps and squats as you can in the two allocated minutes** (to include the original Stand and Thigh Squeeze activity). Use a nearby desk or other piece of furniture if you need assistance squatting down or if balance is somewhat difficult at this point. As you strengthen your legs, both the balance and the tightness in your joints should improve with time. If you have bad knees or hips, alter the squat to accommodate your ability.

The S portion lasts two minutes in its entirety. Your alert system is set up to count down five minutes at a time, so keep an eye on these minutes via the timer or a clock on the wall, and make sure that at approximately two minutes into the five minutes you move on to the next segment, segment L. These approximate allocations of time do not have to be perfect, but make sure the total time for your movement break equals five minutes.

Problem: someone is on the other side of your desk when your alert system sounds. If you were in the middle of a one-on-one meeting right at the moment your alert system goes off, try to find polite reasons why you must stand and simply explain it to the person in front of you. Things like "Oh I'm so sorry but my leg is cramping up, do you mind if I stand a moment? Okay, so you were saying..." and continue the conversation while standing for as long as it is natural and comfortable to do so. Try to remain standing for as long as possible while squeezing the thigh muscles as described above. The person across from you will not know the difference and your business communication can continue without disruption. Tense and flex the rest of your muscles which are all part of the SLAM activity for that five minutes, particularly your abdominal muscles, regardless of whether you choose to sit back down or continue standing. If you do find yourself in a meeting when your alert system sounds, you may have to forego the squats this time, but you can make up for them later in the day. You can do this. You just have to be creative. If for some reason you absolutely must miss one of your SLAM periods, another one will be right behind it to get you back on track, thanks to the schedule you set at the very beginning of your day.

THE L PART OF SLAM: LEGS (TO INCLUDE GLUTES AND HIPS)
After the S segment, return to your chair and sit down. You have three minutes left for movement on the program to complete L, A and M. For Week 1, the leg-exercise list is below **(note: Appendix A provides full descriptions of all SLAM exercises).** Choose one or more of these Leg exercises and repeat them for two minutes. As a reminder, your leg muscles are the biggest muscles in the body, so we are spending more time on the legs via the S and L segments in order to maximize the potential for metabolic processes to kick into gear. The goal is to tax those larger muscles in your body so that they will draw insulin from the blood and decrease chances for diabetes and cancer. You will simultaneously burn calories, which will contribute to your other health goals.

* Simple Knee Lifts
* Simple Leg Extensions
* One-Legged Bicycles

THE A PART OF SLAM: ARMS (TO INCLUDE NECK AND SHOULDERS)
Still seated in your chair, you only have one minute left. You will spend 30 seconds on Arms (plus neck and shoulders) and the other 30 seconds on your Midsection. For the arms, neck and shoulders in Week 1, choose from the following:

* Head turn to the right, hold, then head turn to the left, hold
* Chin to chest, hold, then eyes to ceiling, hold
* Ear to right shoulder, hold, ear to left shoulder, hold

The previous three exercises must finish within 30 seconds. It may seem that looking to the ceiling or shrugging one shoulder at a time might be slightly disruptive or look a bit strange, but in actuality, the movements are brief and can go completely unnoticed.

THE M PART OF SLAM: MIDSECTION (TO INCLUDE THE SPINE)
The final 30 seconds of the five-minute SLAM movement break is for the Midsection and abdominals. Do not worry! This movement is going to remind you that *you have a midsection.*

* Air running with abdominal squeezes for 30 seconds

That is it! Week 1 of your alert system will sound each hour to remind you to move for five minutes at the end of each 60-minute period that you sit at your desk. However, other opportunities are available for you to sneak in some SLAM exercises outside of the alert system. For example, what happens during your restroom and lunch breaks? They do in fact offer more opportunities for incorporating movement into your day. For example:

Restroom-break ideas:
Whenever you are done with your private activities, I would like to suggest that before you leave the stall and/or restroom itself, sneak in a few more SLAM movements **(note: Appendix A provides full descriptions of all SLAM exercises)**, such as:

* S Wall Squats
* L Single-Knee Lifts
* A Standing Pushups
* M Abdominal Squeezes

The confines of a bathroom stall and the greater space of the restroom provide ample space for SLAM exercises. I know that it may sound silly, but the restroom-break exercises can continue throughout your day until bedtime. The truth is that we carry our own personal alert system every time we feel a need to visit the restroom. Once you are "alerted" and once you have used the restroom, take an extra few minutes for some SLAM exercises. Every calorie burned counts for you. Every exercise contributes to more non-exercise activity thermogenesis. *All* natural alert systems, especially hunger, serve as opportunities for us to take breaks. The natural alert system of hunger, which forces a break in your workday, brings us to the topic of your lunch break.

Lunch-break ideas:

Do you eat at your desk for lunch? Try to stop that! The beautiful pause midday provides a rest for your mind and posture relief for your body. Take advantage of the time away from your desk. If the weather permits, take a brisk 20-minute walk, then eat your lunch. If the weather is horrible, walk around the inside of your building or anywhere that gets your metabolic processes moving, but walk for ten minutes before lunch and then walk again for ten minutes after lunch. If you can eat your lunch while standing, that would be ideal. Why? Because you have already been sitting for hours, do you really need to sit more? Have you scheduled a lunch meeting? Sneak in some stealth SLAM movements under the lunch table while discussing business. Incorporate some S (stand), L (one-leg lift two inches off the floor and hold, repeat on other leg), A (palm presses) and M (abdominal squeezes) while seated across from your lunch mate. If walking for 20 minutes during your lunch break does not work for you, start your lunch break with five minutes of SLAM and then finish your lunch break with five minutes of SLAM. Then walk for ten minutes before returning to your desk. The idea is to be cognizant of the need for your body to move and stay in motion, no matter what obstacle impedes your progress. Be creative, find solutions, and empower yourself to take control over your physical existence. Remember, you are not a machine... you are you.

Restroom- and Lunch-Break Ideas

Restroom-Break Suggestions	
Wall Squats	Lean against the bathroom wall or even the wall of the stall if necessary (provided it is stable). Allow your lower back and upper part of your bottom to touch the wall. Do not let your upper back touch the wall. Bend your knees and slide down and then back up again very slowly ten times. Try to squat down far enough, using the wall for stability, to bring your legs to 90 degree angles before rising up.
Single-Knee Lifts	While keeping your balance with hands on hips, lift your right knee to hip height and then slowly lower it, repeating this motion ten times. Do the same with your left knee, also ten times.
Standing Pushups	Bring your feet out away from the bathroom wall approximately two feet, (you may use the stall wall if it is secure) and then place your hands against the wall at chest height. Slowly bring your nose to the wall between your hands and then extend your arms straight. Repeat this motion ten times.
Standing Abdominal Squeezes	While walking back to your desk, pull in your abdominals until they actually hurt. Hold them in as long as you can while you are walking. Release, and then repeat the abdominal pull for as long as it takes to reach your desk.
Lunch-Break Suggestions	Push yourself to find a way to make this break in your day count to your best advantage. FIND A WAY, no matter what,

	to walk for 20 minutes during your lunch break. You might walk ten minutes to a restaurant, dine, and then walk ten minutes back to your desk. You could walk for 20 minutes and then return to eat a lunch that you brought to work. Either way, walk for 20 minutes midday; it will make a world of difference in how the rest of the afternoon goes.
SLAM AT THE LUNCH TABLE:	
Stand	STAND. Tense and squeeze both thigh muscles for a few seconds, then release those muscles. Next, place the majority of your weight on the right leg and squeeze the right thigh muscle. Repeat the same on the left leg.
One-at-a-time Leg Lift	Lift your right leg off the floor two inches. Hold that leg in the air for as long as you can until the burn is intolerable. Repeat with the left leg. You could do this movement for the entire lunch and your lunch partner would never know that you were exercising. Stealth!
Palm Presses (to be done after you eat while you are waiting for the check)	With both feet on the floor, place the palms of your hands together, then press and hold for as long as you can. Repeat as many times through lunch as you can while your hands are free if you are simply conversing.
Abdominal Squeezes	Pull in your abdominal muscles and hold for as long as you can. Release and repeat this movement as many times as you can in between bites of food.

-Week 2

Congratulations! You are beginning your second week on the program. Before you proceed, however, you must first adjust your timer to reflect the increased activity of Week 2. Per the instructions on Page 30, increase the frequency of alerts to every 30 minutes, or twice each hour. We will introduce new exercises in Week 2 and strengthen the habits learned in Week 1.

Once the Interval Timer is set and subsequently sends an alert tone of your choosing, each five-minute movement break consists of the SLAM order of exercises.

For the SLAM order, each segment receives the following time allotment (identical to that of Week 1):

- **S** Stand (steps, squats) = **2 minutes**
- **L** Legs (glutes, hips) = **2 minutes**
- **A** Arms (neck, shoulders) = **30 seconds**
- **M** Midsection (spine) = **30 seconds**

Now, the exercises!

Week 2 continues the commitment to the alert system via the *Office Fitness Fix* Interval Timer app and provides new SLAM exercises. Keep in mind that these are ideas that you may take and expand upon, depending on your levels of creativity and capability. Also remember that ***Appendix A provides full descriptions of all SLAM exercises.***

The S Part Of Slam Week 2: Standing (To Include Steps And Squats)
As mentioned earlier, the S portion of the SLAM exercises are the same in Week 2 as they were in Week 1. Each time your alert goes off (indicating that it is time to get off that chair) IMMEDIATELY STAND. Tense and squeeze both thigh muscles until they burn, then release those muscles. Next, place the majority of your weight on the right leg and squeeze the right thigh muscle. Repeat the same on the left leg.

As in Week 1, your goal for Week 2 is to take some steps and squat down as many times as you can comfortably, physically and discreetly. I mention the word "discreet" quite often in this book, but not because you should feel embarrassed by the fact that you are taking care of yourself. On the contrary, self-care should always be a celebration. The workplace, however, can be a strange environment. If one of the co-workers within an office situation started doing pushups in the middle of the floor, it would seem completely out of place and unprofessional in most offices. For this reason, the *Office Fitness Fix* program encourages a private relationship between you and your health. Making an exercising spectacle of yourself is not the goal here.

Nevertheless, let us get back to those squats. Look around your office. There are ways within your office environment that will allow you to naturally squat down to achieve a professional goal, and do as many squats as possible. Remember the suggestions from Week 1?

- Squat down and reach for something under your desk, using your desk for support if necessary.
- Open and close the bottom drawer of a file cabinet to look for a particular file. (You might in fact want to put your most critical files in that drawer so that you will always have a reason to squat down to obtain them).
- Check the paper supply of the bottom drawer of your copy machine.

You might add to that some other ideas that you found in your own office, such as

- Secure a computer cord at the outlet connection
- Drop your pen or pencil by accident and pick it up

Regardless of the creative ideas you find to squat down in your office, the goal is to **take as many steps and squats as you can in the two allocated minutes** (which includes the original Stand and Thigh Squeeze activity).

As a reminder, your alert system is set up to count down five minutes at a time, so keep an eye on the timer or clock on the wall, and make sure that at approximately two minutes into the five minutes you move on to the next segment, segment L.

THE L PART OF SLAM WEEK 2: LEGS (TO INCLUDE GLUTES AND HIPS)

As in Week 1, return to your chair and sit down after the S portion of the exercises. You have three minutes left for movement on the program to complete L, A, and M. For Week 2, the Leg exercise list is as follows. Choose one or more of these Leg exercises and repeat them for two minutes (descriptions in Appendix A):

* Knee Fans
* Crossed-Ankle Knee Lifts
* Thigh/Knee Squeezes

THE A PART OF SLAM WEEK 2: ARMS (TO INCLUDE NECK AND SHOULDERS)

Still seated in your chair, you only have one minute left. You will spend half of that minute on Arms and the other half on your Midsection. For the arms, neck, and shoulders in Week 2, choose from the following:

* Faux Body Lifts
* Palm presses
* Neck Rolls

THE M PART OF SLAM WEEK 2: MIDSECTION (TO INCLUDE THE SPINE)

The last 30 seconds of the five-minute SLAM movement break is for the abdominal midsection. This is quick, but it will make you feel great!

* Abdominal Squeeze plus Leg Lifts

That is it! Week 2 has your alert system sound twice each hour to remind you to move for five minutes (every 30 minutes you sit at your desk). In addition to these scheduled movement breaks, **be sure to remember the opportunities you have for exercise during your restroom breaks and lunch breaks.**

-WEEK 3

You are halfway through the program as described in this book, but the goal is maintain the exercise breaks in your workday for years to come. Week 3 is an excellent time to learn advanced exercises and to begin incorporating *Office Fitness Fix* Fuel (Chapter 5) recipes and ideas into your day. This is the rare time in the book where I actually encourage you to jump ahead. Since you are on Week 3 and are clearly devoted to the concept of moving while working, reward yourself by reading the *Office Fitness Fix* Fuel section in Chapter 5. These healthful suggestions can improve your dietary intake and encourage you to bring a nutritious selection of foods to the office. Office Fitness Fix Fuel provides information on healthy foods and is especially easy if you join the *Office Fitness Fix* Community. Work-friendly snack and lunch recipes (sent via email) provide inspiration for healthy eating to every member of the Community.

Before you proceed, however, you must first adjust your timer to reflect the increased activity of Week 3. Per the instructions on Page 30, increase the frequency of alerts to every 20 minutes, or three times each hour. We will introduce new exercises in Week 3 and strengthen the habits learned in Weeks 1 and 2.

Again, the Interval Timer is set and subsequently alerts you to perform each five-minute movement break, all consisting of the SLAM order of exercises.

For the SLAM order, each segment receives the following time allotmen (identical to those of Weeks 1 and 2):

S   Stand (steps, squats) = **2 minutes**
L   Legs (glutes, hips) = **2 minutes**

A Arms (neck, shoulders) = **30 seconds**
M Midsection (spine) = **30 seconds**

THE S PART OF SLAM WEEK 3: STANDING (TO INCLUDE STEPS AND SQUATS)
Proceed with the S portion of the SLAM exercises in Week 3 as you did in Weeks 1 and 2. When you hear your alert, immediately stand. Tense and squeeze both thigh muscles until you feel the burn, then relax those muscles. Next, place the majority of your weight on the right leg and squeeze the right thigh muscle. Repeat the same on the left leg.

Now you have another full minute to step and squat as many times as you can muster (without looking strange). Do you need more ideas for getting away with squatting at work? How about the following:

- Bookshelves in your office? Squat down to choose a book on the bottom shelf.
- Are there plants in your office? Relocate a few of them to floor stands, then squat down to water them.
- Locate your office supplies on the bottom shelf or drawer in the office-supply area of your workspace. Squat down to grab some pencils, one at a time; suddenly you need five pencils!

After two minutes spent on S, move to the L exercises.

THE L PART OF SLAM WEEK 3: LEGS (TO INCLUDE GLUTES AND HIPS)
After the S segment, return to your chair and sit down. You have three minutes left for movement on the program to complete L, A and M. For Week 3, the two-minute Leg-exercise list is as follows. Choose one or more of these Leg exercises and repeat them for two minutes. Again, your leg muscles are the biggest muscles in the body, so we are spending more time on the legs via the S and L segments in order to maximize the potential for metabolic processes to kick into gear (exercises fully described in Appendix A):

* Knee Circles
* Air Walking
* Double-Leg Extensions

THE A PART OF SLAM WEEK 3: ARMS (TO INCLUDE NECK AND SHOULDERS)
Still seated in your chair, you only have one minute left. You will spend half of that minute on Arms and the other half on your Midsection. For the arms, neck and shoulders in Week 3, choose from the following:

* High Stress Pull-Aparts
* The Swivel

THE M PART OF SLAM WEEK 3: MIDSECTION (TO INCLUDE THE SPINE)
The last 30 seconds of the five-minute SLAM movement break is for the abdominal midsection. For Week 3, try the following exercise for your abs:

* Air Belly

Week 3 has your alert system sound three times each hour to remind you to move for five minutes for every 20 minutes you sit at your desk. **Do not forget the restroom breaks and lunch breaks as opportunities to move!**

-WEEK 4

You have made it to the final week of learning and moving via the *Office Fitness Fix* 4-week Method! After Week 4, you may start again with the Week 1 exercises for variety, but remember that from Week 4 forward, your movement breaks should be every 15 minutes per the instructions on Page 30. That may seem like a lot, and it is, but these movement exercises do not disrupt your work and have become second nature since you realize that sitting motionless like a lump is only a whisper from your distant past.

From Week 5 and beyond, your commitment to yourself should be clear, and I truly hope that you will commend yourself for your tenacity and accomplishments. Again, change is hard, but you have made it to Week 4, which is a strong indication that you are making a long-term commitment to your physical and mental health. Remember, you are not a machine like your computer. You are a living, breathing human with many organic processes underneath your skin. Keeping the body alive and flourishing will lead to a much happier future and more productive work life.

Each five-minute movement break consists of the SLAM order of exercises once the *Office Fitness Fix* Interval Timer sends an alert.

For the SLAM order, each segment receives the following time allotment (identical to those of Weeks 1,2 and 3):

S Stand (steps, squats) = **2 minutes**
L Legs (glutes, hips) = **2 minutes**
A Arms (neck, shoulders) = **30 seconds**
M Midsection (spine) = **30 seconds**

THE S PART OF SLAM WEEK 4: STANDING (TO INCLUDE STEPS AND SQUATS)
The S portion of the SLAM exercises is the same in Week 4 as it was in Weeks 1, 2 and 3. IMMEDIATELY STAND. Tense and squeeze both thigh muscles for a few seconds, then release those muscles. Next, place the majority of your weight on the right leg and squeeze the right thigh muscle. Repeat the same on the left leg.

For the next minute, your goal is to take some steps and squat down as many times as you can comfortably, physically and discreetly do. Look around your office. Find ways within your office environment that allow you to squat down naturally to achieve a professional goal. Solutions that are more creative might include:

- Back to the bottom file drawers. If you place the waiting items on top of the file cabinet and then squat down each time for placement in a lower drawer, you can go up and down with your squats with practically every sheet of paper. This is an important exercise.

No matter what creative solutions to the Stand, Step and Squat segment of your movement activity, remember that the goal is to do as many squats as you can within the two minutes remaining after you have completed the original Stand and Thigh Squeeze activity. The S portion lasts two minutes in its entirety. Afterwards, move on to segment L.

THE L PART OF SLAM WEEK 4: LEGS (TO INCLUDE GLUTES AND HIPS)
After the S segment, return to your chair and sit down. You have three minutes left for movement on the program to complete L, A and M. For Week 4, the Leg-exercise list is as follows. Again, all descriptions of the exercises are in Appendix 1 at the end of this chapter. Choose one or more of these Leg exercises and repeat them for two minutes. Your leg muscles are the biggest muscles in the body, so we are spending more time on the legs via the S and L segments in order to maximize the potential for metabolic processes to kick into gear in rapid succession:

- Calf Raises
- Tap and Lift
- Thigh and Glute Squeezes

THE A PART OF SLAM WEEK 4: ARMS (TO INCLUDE NECK AND SHOULDERS)
Still seated in your chair, you only have one minute left. You will spend half of that minute on Arms and the other half on your Midsection. For the arms, neck and shoulders in Week 4, choose from the following:

- Stiff-Arm Pulses
- Reverse Shoulder Rolls

THE M PART OF SLAM WEEK 4: MIDSECTION (TO INCLUDE THE SPINE)
The last 30 seconds of the five-minute SLAM movement break is for the abdominal midsection.

- C-curve spine

That is it! Week 4 has your alert system sound every 15 minutes to remind you to move while you sit at your desk. Although moving every 15 minutes may seem like a lot, the movement of these exercises is subtle and stealth. Work disruption is unnecessary. In fact, the biochemical boost and the stress relief on joints will most likely create a more productive work environment.

The Chart below describes the outcome of the *Office Fitness Fix* 4-week method:*

Week	Hours Committed to Movement	Calories Burned per Day	Top Number of Calories Burned per Week	Calories Burned per Year (50 weeks on program)	Average Pounds Lost at Year End
1	1.25	65-125	625	31,250	8.9
2	2	100-200	1000	50,000	14.3
3	2.4	120-240	1200	60,000	17.14
4	3	150-300	1500	75,000	21.4

*based on the "yellow activity" scale, **Move A Little, Lose A Lot**, James A. Levine, MD, PhD and Selene Yeager*

Some pointers about the movement program:

1. On the STAND, STEP and SQUAT, those squats are key for exercising the large muscles of the legs. Try to do as many as you can in the allocated time because they really get the blood pumping.

2. With the remaining exercises for Legs, Arms and Midsection, really try your hardest to tense and squeeze those muscles until they burn. Your goal is to get the enzymatic processes in your body awake and moving, to fight high sugar levels in your blood.

Sedentary living and prolonged sitting without movement is extremely unhealthy, and once you feel the balance in your body and mind through ongoing self-care, *you will be hooked*. Engaging your body in small bursts throughout each day generates enzymatic activity. Your muscles contract, your blood pumps, oxygen flows. Energy returns to your body and your mind. Continue with the scheduled 15-minute breaks in your work life for the remainder of the year and beyond. If you are concerned about burnout or boredom, look for new ideas for movement exercises and healthy recipes via the *Office Fitness Fix* Community, described in Chapter 5.

APPENDIX ONE
EXERCISE LISTS

Week One	Description
Stand	IMMEDIATELY STAND. Tense and squeeze both thigh muscles for a few seconds, then release those muscles. Next, place the majority of your weight on the right leg and squeeze the right thigh muscle. Repeat with left leg.
Steps, Squats	TAKE AS MANY STEPS AND SQUATS as you can in the two minutes allocated for this exercise.
Legs Simple Knee Lifts	Lift right leg two inches off the floor. Pulse right knee upwards for count of 20. Repeat with left leg.
Simple Leg Extensions	Push chair back so you have enough room to extend your legs. Flex and lift right foot and pulse upward for count of 20. Repeat with left foot.
One-Legged Bicycles	Firmly plant your left foot on the floor for balance. Lift right knee two inches off the floor. Circle right ankle around as if you are peddling a bicycle for count of 20. Repeat with left leg.
Arms Head Turns	Turn head to the right, look over right shoulder, hold for count of 8. Repeat to left side.
Chin to Chest then Ceiling	Stretch back of neck by tucking chin to chest. Let gravity sink your chin into your chest and count to 8. Slowly raise eyes to ceiling and count to 8.
One-Shoulder Shrugs	Tilt head to right and touch ear to right shoulder and hold for count of 2. Repeat to left side for count of 2, then repeat one additional time on both sides.
Mid-section Air-running with Abdominal Squeeze	Tighten abs and hold them as firmly as possible for 30 seconds. While holding in abdominal muscles, lift feet off the floor and pulse knees upwards in a running fashion. Keep holding abs firm and count for 30.

Week Two	Description
Stand	IMMEDIATELY STAND. Tense and squeeze both thigh muscles for a few seconds, then release those muscles. Next, place the majority of your weight on the right leg and squeeze the right thigh muscle. Repeat with left leg.

Steps, Squats	TAKE AS MANY STEPS AND SQUATS as you can in the two minutes allocated for this exercise.
Legs Knee Fans	Press knees together and lift feet two inches off the floor. Spread feet apart while holding knees together and lift the feet outward and upward in a pulsing motion for count of 20.
Cross-Ankle Knee Lifts	Cross right ankle over left ankle. Lift right knee up while keeping the ankles in vertical alignment. Pulse the right knee upward for a count of 20. Repeat crossing left ankle over right.
Thigh/Knee Squeezes and Hold	Firmly plant your feet together. With as much strength as you can muster, squeeze your knees together at the same time as you press your ankles together for a count of 20.
Arms Faux Body Lifts	With your palms under your thighs, straighten your arms to simulate "lifting" your body off the chair. Repeat eight times.
Palm Presses	Place both feet on the floor. Place the palms of your hands together, then press and hold for as long as you can. Release. Repeat, counting to 8 each time as you press and hold.
Neck Rolls	Tilt your head to the right and touch your ear to your right shoulder. Roll your head around backwards and return to the starting position for count of 8. Repeat in the opposite direction.
Mid-section Abdominal Squeezes plus Leg Lifts	While seated, tighten abs and hold them as firmly as possible for 30 seconds. While holding in your abdominal muscles, lift your feet off the floor and pulse knees upwards for a count of 30 with knees pressed together. Pull the abdominal muscles in as tight as you can throughout the count of 30.

Week Three	Description
Stand	IMMEDIATELY STAND. Tense and squeeze both thigh muscles for a few seconds, then release those muscles. Next, place the majority of your weight on the right leg and squeeze the right thigh muscle. Repeat on the left leg.

Steps, Squats	TAKE AS MANY STEPS AND SQUATS as you can in the two minutes allocated for this exercise.
Legs Knee Circles	Lift your right leg two inches off the floor. Let your foot hang loosely. Place your arms on your chair for stability so that you can isolate the knee, hip and thigh area. Make slow circles with your right knee in a clockwise direction for a count of ten, then in a counterclockwise direction for a count of ten. Repeat with the left knee.
Air Walking	Lift both feet off the floor and press your knees together. Place your hands on your chair for stability. Holding your knees firm and lifted, "stride" with your feet as if you are walking. Continue this motion for a count of 30. If you are doing this correctly, your thighs should burn by the end of the exercise.
Double-Leg Extensions	Push your chair back a bit to make room for leg extensions under your desk. Slide your bottom to the very back of your chair. Flex your feet so that your toes are pointing toward your midsection. Press your thighs and ankles together and force your heels away from you. Slowly lift both legs simultaneously to a full extension (if you have room). Lower your feet to the floor and repeat 20 times.
Arms High Stress Pull Aparts	Interlock your fingers, flare your elbows outward, using all of your arm strength, and try to pull your hands apart for a slow count of 15. Your upper arms should burn upon completion.
The Swivels	Plant your feet firmly on the floor. Grab the right side of your chair (or the arm of your chair) with both hands. Try to keep your body from the waist down facing forward. Simultaneously, twist the upper half of your body as far to the right as possible, looking over your right shoulder for a count of 15. Repeat on the left side.
Mid-section Air Belly	Sit up straight with your feet planted firmly on the floor. Breathe in through your mouth and try to direct the air to your belly instead of your lungs. Hold your breath and press your

	abdominals outward. Push your stomach outward. Next, pull your abdominals in, exhale, then hold the tightened abs for as long as you can. Repeat three times.

Week Four	Description
Stand	IMMEDIATELY STAND. Tense and squeeze both thigh muscles for a few seconds, then release those muscles. Next, place the majority of your weight on the right leg and squeeze the right thigh muscle. Repeat on the left leg.
Steps, Squats	TAKE AS MANY STEPS AND SQUATS as you can in the two minutes allocated for this exercise.
Legs Calf Raises	Sit up straight with your feet planted firmly on the floor. Raise your heels as high as they will go and then lower your heels back to the floor. This seems easy, but the exercise requires a repeat performance 30 times over. By the count of 30, your ankles will be burning.
Tap and Lift	Sit up straight with your feet planted firmly on floor. Lift your right heel and tap the toe of your right foot on the floor. Use that toe-tap as a springboard for the knee to raise three inches, lifting the entire foot off the floor. Return your foot to the floor and lower your heel. Continue this movement on the right foot for a count of 20. Try to make this entire motion fluid and quick. Repeat on the left side.
Thigh and Glute Squeeze	Move your chair (with you on it) as close to your desk as you can. Lift your right leg off the floor two inches. Bring your ankle backwards as if you are trying to touch your ankle to your bottom with your toes pointed. Flex your thigh and glute muscles for a count of 10 while pushing your ankle higher to the underneath part of the chair. Repeat on the left side. My legs shake when I do this one! You must really squeeze the muscles to make the exercise effective.
Arms Stiff-Arm Pulses	Place your hands at the sides of your thighs. Keep your arms as straight as boards, lifting your body slightly until you rise a bit from your

	chair, then bend your elbows in a pulsing motion. Repeat for a quick count of 20.
Reverse Shoulder Rolls	Sit upright with your feet on the floor and your hands on your lap. Push your shoulders back without sticking your chest out. This move is about the shoulders, not about the chest. Hold your shoulders back for a count of five and then slowly roll your shoulders forward while counting six, seven, eight, nine and ten. Repeat. This one offers relief to tight shoulders and neck.
Mid-section C-Curve Spine	Tighten your abs and hold them as firmly as possible for 30 seconds. While holding in abdominal muscles, curl body downward to make a C-shape of the spine. Keep your abs tight, and then slowly straighten your spine. Repeat the motion for a count of 30.

SLAM FOLLOWING A RESTROOM VISIT/LUNCH	
Restroom-Break Suggestions Wall Squats	Lean against the bathroom wall or even the wall of the stall if necessary (provided it is stable). Allow your lower back and the upper part of your bottom touch the wall. Do not let your back touch the wall. Bend your knees and slide down and then back up very slowly ten times.
Single-Knee Lifts	While keeping your balance with your hands on your hips, lift your right knee to hip height and then slowly lower it, repeating this motion ten times. Repeat on the left side.
Standing Pushups	Bring your feet out from the bathroom wall approximately two feet, (you may use the stall wall if it is secure) and place your hands against the wall at chest height. Slowly bring your nose to the wall between your hands and then extend your arms straight. Repeat this motion ten times.
Standing Abdominal Squeezes	While walking back to your desk, pull in your abdominals until they actually hurt. Hold them in as long as you can while you are walking. Release and repeat the abdominal pull for as long as it takes you to reach your desk.

Lunch-Break Suggestions	Push yourself to find a way to make this break in your day count to your best advantage. FIND A WAY, no matter what, to walk for 20 minutes during your lunch break. You might walk ten minutes to a restaurant, dine, and then walk ten minutes back to your desk. You could walk for 20 minutes and then return to eat a lunch that you brought to work. Either way, walk for 20 minutes midday; it will make a world of difference in how the rest of the afternoon goes.
SLAM AT THE LUNCH TABLE:	
Stand	STAND. Tense and squeeze both thigh muscles for a few seconds, then release those muscles. Next, place the majority of your weight on the right leg and squeeze the right thigh muscle. Repeat on the left side.
One-at-a-time Leg Lifts	Lift your right leg off the floor two inches. Hold that leg in the air for as long as you can until the burn is intolerable. Repeat with the left leg. You could do this movement for the entire lunch and your lunch partner would never know that you were exercising. Stealth!
Palm Presses (to be done after you eat while you are waiting for the check)	Place both feet on the floor. Place the palms of your hands together, then press and hold for as long as you can. Repeat as many times as possible.
Abdominal Squeezes	Pull in your abdominal muscles and hold for as long as you can. Release and repeat this movement as many times as you can in between bites of food.

CHAPTER 5

The Long-Term Commitment: "Hang Out With Eagles"

◆ ◆ ◆

-OFFICE FITNESS FIX FUEL

OFFICE FITNESS FIX IS ABOUT moderation and gradual change toward good habits. It makes sense, then, that the *Office Fitness Fix* Fuel section on dietary advice is much the same. Up to this point, the problems and likely outcomes of a sedentary work life set the stage for a movement solution to counteract the risk. The first three sections of this book reference "calories out." In contrast, the *Office Fitness Fix* Fuel section addresses "calories in." What are you eating? To be more specific, what are you eating during your workday?

In June 2015, the Food and Drug Administration detailed its three-year plan to phase out trans fat throughout the food industry. The reduction of partially hydrogenated oils in foods works in concert with the government's goal to prevent cardiovascular disease and improved public health.

This is great news. People need healthier options in the grocery store and in restaurants, and the FDA, through legislation, supports that quest. "Calories in" *matter*. More importantly, the types of calories you consume matter even more. Let us return to the question: what are you eating during your workday? If your workplace provides cookies, cakes and vending machines filled with unhealthy lunch choices, your challenge is great. How in the world can you say no to all of that temptation? There is a way, and you can absolutely battle the seduction of unhealthy food choices.

Our working hours represent a significant part of our day; they are also the part of our day when we are sedentary and a bit trapped. The *Office Fitness Fix* 4-week method encourages you to get *un-trapped* from your desk. *The Office Fitness Fix* Fuel section describes ways to become *un-trapped* from your diet.

How is this accomplished? Improved food selection is possible in the same way increased movement into your workday is possible: through moderation, gradual change, and the careful development of habits that *stick*.

Just as you slowly adopted more movement over time in Chapter 4, the simultaneous effort of making better food choices should also happen with time. It would be ridiculous for me to create another entry into the flooded diet industry called the *Office Fitness Fix* Diet. Besides, fad diets rarely work in the long term. However, improving the nutritional content of your food intake while keeping an eye on calories is both necessary and achievable. Just as you have made a commitment to health by incorporating movement throughout each workday, now you must address the other half of the equation: *calories in*.

What to eat? I always liked the phrase by Susan Powter in the 1980's when she said, *"If it didn't grow that way, don't eat it."* Admittedly, Susan Powter lost momentum with her listening audience because of her restrictions on healthy fats, but shifting your choices to foods in their natural state is a basic and important change to your diet. Did a chocolate chip muffin grow that way? No, it did not. Did an apple grow that way? You bet it did.

When I arrive at my local coffee shop each morning, I face the gorgeous glass case of croissants, cakes and cookies. I simply and flatly say to myself, "That's not for me." Then I order something I can recognize in its whole form. Many coffee shops offer fruit, salads and nuts. Cheese does not "grow that way," but it is real food and is something to be considered. If you pull yourself away from "fluffy food" with its minimal nutritional value and its rich amount of fat and calories, you begin the slow process of improving the quality of "calories in." Does this mean that you will go to your coffee shop each day for the next week and never order a muffin? I personally think that goal is unrealistic. However, for a couple of days in the first week, you might say, "I had that muffin yesterday, I'll order the cheese and fruit plate today," and then you will be well on your way to shifting old habits. This kind of shift, the one toward real food and away from food with little nutritional value, is one that has the potential to last.

You can especially manage the slow substitution of healthy choices over unhealthy choices in your own work life. You already know what unhealthy foods look like, so while you are following the *Office Fitness Fix* method of movement, design a plan for yourself where you begin the process of replacing unhealthy food choices that you typically consume during office hours. For example, you might commit to replacing unhealthy snacks or meals just once a day in Week 1, and then twice a day in Week 2, and so on. This gradual adoption of healthier eating habits over time rewards you without the awful feeling of deprivation. The slow shift toward better food choices also sidesteps the worst part of dieting: hunger. Eat already! Just make the transition to real, whole food. If the vending machine temptations are great, buy something each morning in its whole form elsewhere and avoid the vending machine altogether. You are spending money either way, but spending your money on foods in their natural state builds the arsenal to fight for health and weight control.

I had a sweet tooth in my younger days. I adored sweets, especially birthday cake from a bakery with its white, fat-filled, sugary icing. Once I made the commitment to consume most foods in their natural state, (I am not perfect at this, and I still work on it), I became so satisfied via the fiber and nutrients in the whole food that "fluffy food" no longer had an appeal. In fact, at those times when I chose to accept the gracious offer of cake at a birthday celebration, I felt as though I had Crisco on my teeth and glue in my stomach. Yuck! The more you consume whole foods, the less you will want to waste your time on empty calories. Food is fuel.

> "I never worry about diets. The only carrots that interest me are the number you get in a diamond."
>
> -Mae West

You may choose to ignore a recommended change in your diet, just like Mae West; you may also choose to rely solely on *the Office Fitness Fix* 4-week movement method. However, weight loss is not the only goal here. The goal is improved health. The goal is warding off serious illness, feeling better and having more energy. Better eating habits positively contribute to each of those goals.

Need more support with your diet? The *Office Fitness Fit* Community might be something that you should consider. Through the Community, ongoing support strengthens your resolve and therefore your commitment to health.

-Office Fitness Fix Community

Why join a community to help you in your quest toward health? In 2013, Baylor College of Medicine reported its findings following a 292-person randomized trial with the conclusion that "a community-based approach to weight loss yielded significantly greater results compared to the self-help approach." Being part of the *Office Fitness Fix* Community offers the same type of systemic support.

Through a low-cost membership ($4.99 per month, a little over a dollar each week), weekly emails will help you stay motivated and on track with the *Office Fitness Fix* program and your diet. Each newsletter will contain the following:

* FUEL- Delicious and healthy recipes for ongoing snack and meal swaps (unhealthy fluff to healthy whole-food nutrition)
* FITNESS- New stealth SLAM exercises to try and reviews of advanced exercise equipment available for your office or home, with links for purchase
* FUN- Upbeat music suggestions for your 20-minute walk during lunchtime
* FASHION- Office fashion inspiration for a comfortable yet professional wardrobe for men and women
* FACTS and FAQs

With regard to the healthy recipes, I continually search for the best recipes and ideas for healthy eating at work that are realistic and doable. The goal is to take these recipes one at a time, and slowly incorporate them into your reality. Make these recipes at home the night before, make extra, and bring the leftovers to work the next day in a lunchbox. (If you eat out the night before, order an extra hearty salad "to go" and carry that healthy food choice to work the next day.) If you do nothing else but bring one healthy food option as a substitute for an on-the-fly lunch option this week, you are beginning the gradual change toward healthier eating habits.

What does the Community provide you in the realm of new exercise ideas? Creativity! Stealth exercising at your desk limits a movement explosion (so not to disrupt workflow), but there are many muscles in our bodies that wait to be challenged and utilized. We wish to touch every single one of them.

The Community offers analysis of and ordering information for advanced exercise equipment. At your desk? In your office? You bet. By adding exercise bands, yoga sandbags and exercise balls, the *Office Fitness Fix* movement breaks expand to a new level of stealth, while remaining discreet. Those lucky ones with private offices, or the professionals who work from home, can learn important information about under-the-desk elliptical machines, hand weights, and even treadmill desks via the Community weekly email.

Your lunchtime walks restore your human energy and stimulate your brain cells. Rather than slump behind your computer with another four hours to go, you will return to your desk energized and ready to work. Adding upbeat music to that walk makes it enjoyable! If you sometimes get lost in the iTunes marketplace (or other music platform), the weekly emails from the Community will provide you with new songs to add zip to your pace and zing to your energy.

Now to the topic involving the most creativity -- fashion! In many offices, the professional wardrobe has relaxed a bit. This trend spawned the new term "athleisure," a combination of "athletics" and "leisure-wear" that has become a billion-dollar industry. Professional women now wear high-quality "dress yoga pants" with tailored cardigan sets and appropriate jewelry; professional men wear charcoal-gray "dress sweatpants" that look like business wear but feel as comfortable as sweats. Talk about win-win! How much more productive would you be if you were actually *comfortable* in that chair all day long? The Community newsletter will keep you on top of the trend with links to professional athleisure-wear websites.

"If you hang out with chickens, you're going to cluck.
If you hang out with eagles, you're going to soar."

–Dr. Steve Maraboli

Joining the *Office Fitness Fix* Community surrounds you with ideas, inspiration and suggestions from other professionals who strive to achieve the same goals. You may join the Community by visiting www.officefitnessfix.com and clicking on the "Join the Community" link.

For many professionals, the position they hold at work somewhat defines them. In truth, however, we all are individuals with our own goals, aspirations, hang-ups, insecurities, strengths and passions. We define our individual selves, but sometimes that individuality can get lonely. We are born naked and alone, and we die naked and alone, but that journey in the middle includes friends, partners, kids, pets, colleagues and bosses who sustain us. Community sustains us and keeps us on track.

For the blessing of your individual self and your community, strive to take care of the body you inhabit. Dig deep to fuel that body in an efficient way. Entertain that body with music, sights and tastes that bring you joy. Decorate that body with clothes that comfort and soothe you. Life allows you to enjoy your own creativity and to be proud of what you bring to the table. If you must work at a desk in order to make a living, enjoy it, and be well in your work life.

A Special Note To Employers:

◆ ◆ ◆

IN OCTOBER 2014, A MULTI-CENTER study in Spain, Australia and the United Kingdom confirmed the direct association between the sitting time of office employees and their productivity and mental well-being. The conclusion stressed that "workplace physical-activity strategies to improve the mental well-being and productivity of all employees should focus on reducing sitting time alongside efforts to increase physical activity."[13]

Encouraging desk-based movement exercises along with standing breaks and "walking meetings in motion" are just a few inexpensive and safe ways to increase productivity and employee health. Business productivity increases in direct proportion to employee wellness; similarly, executing a strategy to foster movement in the workplace allows for greater project-completion rates and highly-engaged employees. Both the employee and the employer benefit greatly by movement campaigns in the workplace.

FOOTNOTES

1. The Bureau of Labor Statistics, American Time Use Survey. http://www.bls.gov/TUS/CHARTS/home.html.

2. The World Health Organization, Fact Sheet No 385, Updated January 2015. http://www.who.int/mediacentre/factsheets/fs385/en/

3. McDermott, Melissa "Sitting for Long Periods Increases Risk of Disease and Death, Regardless of Exercise." Press Release from UH Toronto Rehabilitation Institute. January 19, 2015 http://www.uhn.ca/corporate/News/PressReleases/Pages/Sitting_study.aspx

4. AUSDab Study Original Investigation, Mar 26, 2012, "Sitting Time and All-Cause Mortality Risk in 222,497 Australian Adults." Hidde P. van der Ploeg, PhD; Tien Chey, MAppStats; Rosemary J. Korda, PhD; Emily Banks, MBBS, PhD; Adrian Bauman, MBBS, PhD, Arch Intern Med. 2012;172(6):494-500. doi:10.1001/archinternmed.2011.2174.

5. Berkowitz, Bonnie and Clark, Patterson. "The Health Hazards of Sitting." The Washington Post, Health & Science. January 20, 2014. http://apps.washingtonpost.com/g/page/national/the-health-hazards-of-sitting/750/. Accessed 4.26.151.

6. Watson, Stephanie. "Too Much Sitting Linked to an Early Death." Harvard Health Publications, January 29, 2014. http://www.health.harvard.edu/blog/too-much-sitting-linked-to-an-early-death-201401297004. Accessed 4.26.151.

7. American J. of Clinical Nutrition, April, 2010 and Archives of Internal Medicine, May 2010 and Dr. Gabe Mirkin http://drmirkin.com/fitness/dangers-of-prolonged-sitting.html.

8. Journal of the National Cancer Institute, Dr. Graham Colditz http://jnci.oxfordjournals.org/content/106/7/dju098.abstract

9. Boyle, Terry, Western Institute for Medical Research, University of Western Australia "Long-Term Sedentary Work and the Risk of Subsite-specific Colorectal Cancer." Report from the American Journal of Epidemiology. December 22, 2010 http://aje.oxfordjournals.org/content/173/10/1183

10. Joan Vernikos, M.D., *Sitting Kills, Moving Heals*, Fresno California, Quill Driver Books, 2011

11. Shoham N, Gottlieb R, Shaharabani-Yosef O, et al. Tel Aviv University, "Static Mechanical Stretching Accelerates Lipid Production in 3T3-L1 Adipocytes by Activating the MEK Signaling Pathway." American Journal of Physiology – Cell Physiology. September 27 2011

12. James A. Levine, M.D. Ph.D., *Get Up! Why Your Chair is Killing You and What You Can Do About It*, New York, NY, Palgrave MacMillan, 2014, and *Move a Little, Lose A Lot: How NEAT Science Reveals How to Be Thinner, Happier, and Smarter*, New York, NY, Three Rivers Press, 2009.

13. "Self-reported sitting time and physical activity: interactive associations with mental well-being and productivity in office employees." *BMC Public Health* 2015, 15:72 doi:10.1186/s12889-015-1447-5, http://www.biomedcentral.com/1471-2458/15/72

* 9 7 8 0 6 9 2 4 5 1 5 9 5 *